AF499457

Contents

Newlywed Cooking....................................6

Kitchen Basics Every Newlywed Couple Needs...7

How to Meal Plan with Your Partner Without Fighting..16

ADDITIONAL TIPS TO HELP YOU START MEAL PLANNING FOR TWO:..................................24

The Top 6 Healthy Habits For Newlywed.........28

The Essential Newlywed Home Grocery Shopping List..31

Newlywed Home Grocery List: Paper Items and Cleaning Supplies 31

New Home Grocery List: Fresh Food Essentials 34

Newlywed Home Grocery List: Basic Kitchen Staples..39

Newlywed Home Grocery List: Spice It Up ...45

Newlywed Home Grocery List: Personal Items 49

NEWLYWED RECIPES 51

LEMON AND GARLIC ROAST CHICKEN...........51

Cauliflower Alfredo Sauce with Spaghetti 55

Stuffed French Toast......................................59

2-Hour Turkey...62

Best Fudge Brownie Mix 67

Marmalade Cream Cheese Coffee Cake 69

Hamburger, Sausage, Broccoli Alfredo - Low Carb 74

Yummy Chicken 77

Eggplant Parmesan..79

5 Cheese Macaroni 83

Cream Cheese Stuffed Shells 86

The Original "Easiest Pineapple Cake" 89

Twice Baked Potato Casserole 91

Roast Sticky Chicken Rotisserie Style Like the Deli...94

My Favorite Loaded Potato Soup....................97

Hearty Lasagna for Two.............................100

Quinoa Stuffed Mushrooms.........................107

Enchilada Stuffed Shells 113

Crock Pot Cheesy Scalloped Potatoes and Ham 117

Chicken Alfredo 121

Biscuits & Gravy Breakfast Casserole 123

Amazing "Date Night" Chicken Tacos 126

Warm Ya up Chili..130

Deli Roses 133

London Broil 135

Crunchy Schnitzel with Veggie Chips 137

Asian Beef Stir Fry Bowl Asian Beef Stir Fry Bowl

.... 142

Easy Teriyaki Salmon 145

Broccoli Mini Kugels 147

Oven Fried Cornflake Chicken 148

Newlywed Cooking

Cooking is a skill that improves with experience. Those famous chefs you've heard about either went to culinary school for many years or have just been cooking and perfecting on their own for a while.

Yet, that is not usually the case for newlyweds. Many new couples find themselves stumped when, after many tense and tiring weeks of wedding prep, they settle into their new lives and find a new source of daily stress: Dinner.

We're here to help. Even though it may seem intimidating at first, these easy and basic recipes will allow you to slowly enter the fun and creative world of cooking – and, cook delicious, hearty dinners for each other, too!

Happy cooking!

Kitchen Basics Every Newlywed Couple Needs

You may have spent your entire dating life eating out for every. single. meal, but trust us: the moment you tie the knot, nesting mode totally kicks in. That means saying goodbye to those nightly meet-ups at your fave restaurant and hello to home-cooked goodness in your new dining room.

1. A Tea Pot

Every fabulous morning starts with a nice cup of tea or coffee, so investing in a really great tea pot is definitely key. Plus, they always make your kitchen look so, so pretty. pop of color.

2. A Utensil Set

You can keep digging around in every drawer for the right spoon, or you can register for a utensil set that will make everything that much easier. We vote the latter.

3. A Utensil Crock

Once you have those utensils, you'll need a place to store them and when it comes to choosing a utensil crock, the prettier, the better. (It will sit on your counter, after all.)

And as long as we're finding the perfect spot to store your utensils, let's add in a spoon rest, too.

You'll never realize how much you needed one until you have it.

5. A Coffee Pot

We probably don't need to tell you why this is important, because, well... coffee makes the world go 'round. We're all for registering for an amazing coffee pot, so you and your love can take time to catch up in the am, rather than standing in line at the coffee stand. Our pick? This Cuisinart beauty is programmable, so you'll have a fresh cup of jo waiting every. single. Morning.

6. A Canister Set

Whether you've been baking your heart out since forever, or you're just getting started, a great canister set makes all of the difference. It keeps that sugar, flour, etc. handy while whipping up that banana bread AND makes a pretty statement piece, to boot.

7. Measuring Cups

These might not be glamorous, but if you've been using a drinking cup to measure out your ingredients (been there, done that), it's time to register for the real deal. Our pick? These Le Creuset beauts are so professional, you should have your own tv show.

8. Measuring Spoons

Ditto on the above, but this time with a table spoon. Our pick? This set is sleek AND stainless steel, so you can't go wrong.

9. An Oven Mitt and Potholder

We're big fans of a cute oven mitt and potholder set, because they always, always come in handy and are also a super sweet addition to your kitchen.

10. A Dutch Oven

From cooking up roasts to baking up your fave dessert, a dutch oven will quickly become your go-to for all things in the kitchen. Registering for one of these babies is basically a must - and you'll love the versatility it gives you for all of those dinner parties you and your love will be hosting. Our pick? The Le Creuset Cast Iron Dutch Oven, of course.

11. A Vase

We obviously believe that no room in the house is complete without a beautiful arrangement of flowers, and the kitchen is certainly no exception. Try it - it's like a little ray of sunshine every morning. Our pick? This kate spade beauty from Wayfair for its simple, yet lovely aesthetic.

12. A Cutting Board

You can't have breakfast or brunch without a side of fresh fruit, so we're all for finding the perfect cutting board to get you through every meal with ease.

13. A Knife Set

Newlywed life means giving away those mismatched cutlery item and really investing in some pieces that will last a lifetime. Our pick?

This stainless steel set from Wusthof for its easy grip and maintainability.

14. A Serving Tray

Once you slice up those yummy treats, you need a cute way to serve them, because finding an amazing serving tray is always the first step to impressing your guests. Our pick? You can't go wrong with pineapples, you guys, and this Lenox piece is all sorts of fun.

15. Kitchen Towels

It's the little things that make a difference and having durable towels on hand will make everything that much easier in the kitchen. Bonus points if they're absolutely stunning.

16. A Pan Set

No one tells you just how amazing a "real" pan set can be, so we're letting you in on the secret: scrap those mismatched ones from college and register for the real deal. Your kitchen life will change for the better, we promise. Our pick? This 5-piece stainless steel pan set from Wayfair is giving us all the feels.

17. Jar Candle

Seems simple, but once you create that amazing meal, you'll want to set the mood with a little candlelight and a sweet scent filling your abode. Which means you'll need some candles..

18. Salt Cellar

It's one of those things you didn't know you needed until you can't live without it, but trust us on this one: a salt cellar will streamline your cooking life in ways you didn't think possible.

19. Lazy Susan

We know what you're thinking - a Lazy Susan is for your parents. But you honestly couldn't be more wrong. Add this to your registry for a convenient way to pass the condiments at dinner, or a beautiful centerpiece in your kitchen for herbs and such.

20. Salt & Pepper Shaker

It's back to the basics with two tools you most certainly can't do without - salt and pepper shakers. But don't just grab a couple from the grocery store - we suggest registering for a pretty duo that will really impress your guests.

How to Meal Plan with Your Partner Without Fighting

We all know the benefits of meal planning. Whether you've read about them or heard about them from your friends, you've gotten the gist — planning your meals ahead of time can streamline your budget, make grocery shopping more efficient, save you hassle on chaotic weekdays, and help you eat healthier. There are a lot of upsides.

Meal planning isn't without its stresses, though, especially if you're doing it with a partner. You and your significant other may not agree on the foods you should be eating, the amount of money you should be spending on them, or how often you should be eating in versus going out. It should hardly come as a surprise, then, that meal planning can cause tension in a relationship.

To save you arguments and keep you on track with those meal plans. These are the best advice on meal planning with a partner.

1. Make a master list of meals to choose from.

If you and your partner find the prospect of meal planning totally overwhelming, you probably just avoid it. Sometimes, all you need is a good (and easy) place to start.

Marriage coaches and authors Ashley and Marcus Kusi have a master list that they go back to over and over again. The list includes all of their staple and favorite meals, as well as special things they like to eat for big occasions or holidays. "We can then recycle this list and adjust accordingly every month, saving us time," they say.

Here's how to do it: Create a shared Google doc and brain dump all of the meals that you and/or your partner can make, like to eat, or want to try. If you want to be an overachiever, you can even break the list down into categories based on main ingredients or level of difficulty! Add to the list as you build on your cooking repertoire.

Making the list should be fun and, once you have the list, it will give you starting place to talk through potential menu options together, instead of struggling to remember what your options even are.

2. Be prepared to split the budget.

In your relationship, the stress of meal planning may come down to the bottom line. As you and your partner begin plotting out a weekly menu and building a grocery list, one or both of you might get panicky about the budget, especially if you come at finances with very different perspectives. If that's the case, you may need to get creative with your finances.

"If meal planning and eating specific or more expensive types of food is very important to you, you should personally set aside a larger part of your own budget to cover your special meal plan or — even better! — both your special plan and your partner's plan," life coach and relationship expert Stacy Caprio advises. "It makes [your partner] feel safe and allows you to choose exactly what you want to eat without worrying about the costs."

Here's how to do it: Let's say your partner wants (expensive!) sushi more often than you're willing to splurge on it? Tell him you're in — but it's gotta come from his budget for the week. If you you and your partner share all your finances, this is obviously a bit harder to put into action, but you can sit down to look at your budget and talk about how much you each believe can/should be going toward food. That conversation alone might help you see each other with a better understanding.

3. Respect each other's food stories.

Food is about more than just ingredients on a plate — it's also related to memories, culture, family, body image, health, and so many other things. If you and your partner struggle to get on the same page while you meal plan, it might not actually be about the food at all! There could be more than you realize happening under the surface.

To minimize stress and fighting during meal planning, Caprio emphasizes the importance of respecting your significant other's history with food. Remember that you guys may think about and relate to food differently. "This is a great way to help the other person feel understood, as well as to expand your own food horizons," she says.

Here's how to do it: Take time to talk about why you love taco night so much and why your husband says sandwiches aren't an appropriate dinner. In this way, meal planning can even create opportunities for you and your partner to learn more about each other.

4. Use meal planning as an act of love.

If you're familiar with Gary Chapman's five love languages, you may already be aware that some people receive and express love best through quality time or acts of service. According to marriage and family therapist Amy Rollo, meal planning is as good a time as any for either of those things.

Here's how to do it: Turn a meal planning session into real quality time by turning on your favorite playlist and opening a bottle of wine. Ease your way into the nitty gritty of meal planning by chatting about your other plans for the week first. And then plan to do the cooking part together, too. Are acts of service more your thing? Volunteer to do the grocery shopping and the cooking once you guys settle on a meal plan.

5. Try new recipes.

The Kusis are big believers in the importance of keeping things fresh — both in your relationship and in your joint meal plan. One of their monthly meal planning practices is to have each person choose a new recipe to try.

Making it a habit to experiment with new recipes will keep the meal planning conversation from getting stale and will keep the process interesting so that you'll actually look forward to it. It will also ensure that you have plenty of options to add to your ongoing master list of go-to meals.

ADDITIONAL TIPS TO HELP YOU START MEAL PLANNING FOR TWO:

Set aside a dedicated block of time every weekend. It's preferable to do my meal planning on Sunday mornings, but pick a time and day that works best for your schedule. Keep in mind you'll want to do your grocery shopping after planning your meals for the week, so make sure you meal plan in plenty of time to shop for the week, too. It's preferable to spend about 30 minutes each Sunday jotting down each night's dinner, a list of items to have on hand for breakfast and lunches, and then create a grocery list based off our meals for the week.

Prep your food after grocery shopping. If at all possible, prep any foods for the week you can ahead of time. For instance, wash and dry all your fruits and vegetables, bake any protein you plan to use, and place individual portions of items in Ziploc bags or tupperware to quickly grab for breakfast or lunch.

Take the week's schedule into account. If you know you'll be late returning home on night, plan to have extra leftovers from the night before ready or put your slow cooker to use. This will ensure you're using the food you've paid for and not deciding to order takeout because you're starving and haven't even thought about dinner.

Buy bulk items and prepare them differently throughout the week. Bulk items are often going to be cheaper than smaller quantities. Buy in bulk and prepare the same foods in different ways throughout the week to save money. So you don't get bored with the same foods, switch up which bulk items you get each week.

Plan meals around your coupons. If you're a coupon clipper, check your coupons before planning your meals. Plan meals around the coupons you've clipped to save money on your grocery bill.

Buy what's in season. For produce, stick with items that are currently in season in your area. Seasonal items are much fresher, taste better, and are cheaper than out-of-season produce.

Leave room for leftovers. This is a new tip we've just recently learned after weeks and weeks of meal planning. We found out that couples are wasting money by buying excess food they weren't eating and throwing away. We have leftover food two or three nights a week, so always build in one or two days each week that you don't plan to prepare dinner. On those nights, that there is leftovers turn the leftovers into a new meal. Another option is to have leftovers for lunch and you won't have to plan any lunch items during your meal planning session each week!

The Top 6 Healthy Habits For Newlywed

1. Have "go-to" items that are always in your house for quick meals and snacks. Limit the presence of unhealthy snacks like chips and cookies.

2. Many people complain that they don't like buying fresh fruit or veggies because they go bad before having a chance to use them. While planning out your weekly meals can help limit this, another smart option is buying frozen fruits and veggies. These are picked and frozen at their peak to maintain nutrients, and they can often have a higher nutritional value than those found in the produce section of the market. Frozen items can last longer and be used as

needed. Just avoid buying those items that are frozen along with sauces or heavy syrups.

3. Eat breakfast. This isn't new information, but research has shown on multiple occasions that people who eat breakfast have healthier weights than those who don't. Skipping breakfast can lead to overeating at other meals or grazing throughout the day for people who feel the need to "catch up."

4. Aim to eat every three to four hours, alternating meals with snacks (which are just small meals) to help maintain healthy energy levels and metabolism. This also prevents overeating at meals or causing metabolism to slow down.

5. Plate your meals first, rather than putting the whole serving platter on the table. Additional servings can tempt us if we see them, so simply take them away from your line of sight. Fill your plate with 1/4 lean protein, 1/4 healthy grain or starch, and 1/2 fruit or veggies. And if you make it a goal to have a small salad each night before your main meal, not only are you guaranteeing that you have adequate veggies that day, but you're filling up on healthy veggies, which can limit intake of some higher-calorie foods during the actual meal.

6. Stop eating off your spouse's plate. Those little bites here and there add up over time without you even realizing it's happening. Allow a little to be left behind as a reminder that you don't have to clean your plate at every meal.

The Essential Newlywed Home Grocery Shopping List

The wait is over, but before you can settle in, you're going to need this ultimate newlywed home grocery shopping list! If you check everything off this list, you'll have a fully stocked kitchen ready for summer BBQs, and everything in between. Whether you are just a newlywed or are settling into your first apartment, this grocery list is for you.

While the items on this new home grocery list add up to be a little pricey, purchasing these kitchen staples will make your future grocery shopping trips far less expensive.

Newlywed Home Grocery List: Paper Items and Cleaning Supplies

Whether you love the feeling of clean floors or just want to make sure you can use your dishwasher on the daily, make sure to check these items off your grocery list.

- Toilet paper
- Toilet cleaner
- Toilet brush
- Paper towels
- Napkins
- Tissues
- Trash bags
- Ziploc bags
- Laundry detergent
- Stain remover

- Fabric softener
- Dishwashing soap
- Sponges
- Dishwasher detergent
- Glass cleaner like Windex
- Stainless steel cleaner
- Air freshening spray
- All-purpose cleaner like Lysol or Mr. Clean
- Wood floor cleaner (if necessary)
- Carpet cleaner
- Swiffer with dry and wet pads (or a mop and a bucket)
- Plastic wrap

- Aluminum foil
- Wax paper
- Parchment paper
- Light bulbs

New Home Grocery List: Fresh Food Essentials

Produce

Whether you love eating a wide variety of fruits and vegetables or can only stomach broccoli with a generous dose of butter, make sure to add your favorites to your new home grocery list. Throw some of these fruits and veggies in your shopping cart and you'll find yourself ready to whip up a nutrient-filled dinner in no time!

- Apples
- Oranges
- Bananas
- Clementines
- Lemon
- Lime
- Berries
- Grapes
- Peaches
- Plums
- Avocados
- Tomatoes
- Cucumbers

- Lettuce
- Spinach
- Broccoli
- Asparagus
- Green beans
- Celery
- Carrots
- Potatoes
- Peppers
- Onions

Meats, Fish and Other Proteins

Meat-eaters and seafood lovers, this one's for you. Whether you're feeling fresh salmon or just a classic hamburger, this list has got you covered! Remember not to add too much fresh fish and meat to your grocery list, unless you see yourself cooking within three days of purchase! It's a good idea to stick with longer-lasting frozen meat and fish when you first move-in.

- Eggs
- Deli meats
- Chicken
- Fish
- Shrimp
- Steak
- Ground beef or turkey
- Hot dogs

- Ground sausage

Dairy

Don't forget these dairy items on your grocery list – cereal isn't quite the same without the milk! If you're not a dairy lover, most of these foods can be substituted with a non-dairy alternative.

- Milk
- Butter
- Cream cheese
- Cheese slices
- Yogurt

Bakery

Whether you love your morning toast or really need your favorite cookies to make it through that afternoon slump, be sure to check these items off your list.

- Bread, rolls, pitas, or other sandwich preferences
- Bagels, English muffins, muffins, donuts, or other breakfast preferences
- Cookies, cakes, or other dessert preferences

Newlywed Home Grocery List: Basic Kitchen Staples

Baking Staples

Whether you’re a baking expert or find your cookies consistently burnt, it’s a good idea to have some baking staples on hand. With these items, you'll be prepared to make homemade muffins when the craving calls or simply add some flour to an amazing homemade teriyaki sauce. With these essentials on your grocery list, the possibilities are endless!

- Flour
- Sugar
- Baking soda
- Baking powder
- Yeast
- Vanilla extract
- Shortening
- Chocolate chips

- Breadcrumbs

Frozen Food Essentials

Amidst the chaos of unpacking your first apartment or new home, you're going to want plenty of frozen food on hand. Make sure to add these foods to your new home grocery shopping list, and you'll be ready to prepare a quick, easy, and yummy meal after a long day of unpacking.

Pro shopping tip: Buying frozen fruits and vegetables is a great way to save money — and they'll last longer.

- Vegetables (peas, green beans, carrots, corn, mixed vegetables)
- Fruit (berries, mango, peaches)

- Frozen meat (burgers, chicken nuggets, etc.)
- Pizza
- French fries
- Waffles
- Ice-cream

Cans, Jars, and Boxes

Your first shopping trip after moving into an apartment or house is the perfect time to pick up some canned and jarred items. These pantry gems will stay safe to eat for ages and are the perfect addition to a quick and easy weekday meal. Add these items to your new home grocery list, and you'll be one step closer to a fully stocked kitchen.

- Breakfast cereal
- Rice
- Pasta and/or spaghetti
- Pasta sauce
- Canned soup and/or chili
- Canned beans
- Canned vegetables
- Canned tuna
- Chicken, vegetable, or beef broth

Snack Staples

With all the meal planning you may be doing, you don't want to forget some snacks on your new home grocery list! Of course, you have your favorites, but here are a few items to get you started.

- Snack crackers (Cheez-Its, Goldfish)
- Chips, pretzels, or similar snacks
- Popcorn
- Nuts
- Microwavable snacks (think Bagel Bites, Hot Pockets)

Beverage Central

You might be just fine with tap water. If not, don't forget to add some drinks to your new home grocery list before you get too thirsty!

- Coffee and/or tea

- Bottled water, or water pitcher and filter
- Seltzer water
- Juice
- Soda

Newlywed Home Grocery List: Spice It Up

Spices and Seasonings

Any new home grocery list would be incomplete without spices and seasonings. These items can take just about any dish to the next level, so make sure you check these items off your shopping list—according to your preferences!

- Salt
- Pepper

- Red pepper flakes
- Parsley
- Paprika
- Italian seasoning
- Chili powder
- Cumin
- Basil
- Oregano
- Rosemary
- Dill
- Ginger
- Cinnamon
- Garlic

- Cilantro

Condiments and Sauces

One of the best parts of making a new home grocery list is adding in your favorite sauces and condiments. Whether you want to spice up your weekday dinners and or kick up the heat on your weekend eggs n' bacon, don't neglect these cooking essentials on your first shopping trip.

- Oil (olive, vegetable, canola, sesame, etc.)
- Vinegar (white, balsamic)
- Salad dressings
- Ketchup
- Mustard
- Relish

- Pickles
- Maple syrup
- Honey
- Soy sauce
- Tabasco or sriracha sauce
- Worcestershire sauce
- BBQ sauce
- Steak sauce
- Mayo or Miracle Whip
- Jam or jelly
- Nut butter

Newlywed Home Grocery List: Personal Items

You may already have many of these items on hand. If not, you definitely don't want to neglect the personal care section of your local grocery store. These final items on our new home grocery list will ensure that your bathroom has everything you need to stay clean and look great, too.

- Hand soap
- Deodorant
- Shampoo
- Conditioner
- Bar soap or body wash
- Facial cleaner

- Lotion
- Cotton swabs and balls
- Toothbrush
- Toothpaste
- Dental floss
- Shaving cream
- Feminine products
- Hair styling products
- Razors
- Band-Aids
- Antibiotic ointment
- Anti-inflammatory such as Advil

Once you pick up all the items you need on this ultimate newlywed grocery shopping list, you'll be ready to settle into brand new home.

NEWLYWED RECIPES

These easy and basic recipes will allow you to slowly enter the fun and creative world of cooking – and, cook delicious, hearty dinners for each other, too!

Happy cooking!

LEMON AND GARLIC ROAST CHICKEN

Prepartion time

2 hours 5 minutes

INGREDIENTS

- 2 garlic cloves
- kosher salt
- 1 lemon, halved and juiced, halves reserved
- 1 teaspoon rosemary
- 1 teaspoon sweet paprika
- 3/4 teaspoon ground cumin
- 1/2 teaspoon hot paprika
- fresh ground pepper
- 1/4 cup extra virgin olive oil
- 1 (3 lb) chicken
- 2 tablespoons unsalted butter, softened

Instructions

1. Preheat the oven to 350.

2. On a work surface, mince the garlic with 1 teaspoon of kosher salt.

3. Transfer the garlic to a small bowl and whisk in the lemon juice, rosemary, sweet paprika, cumin, and 1/2 teaspoon pepper, whisk in the olive oil.

4. Using your fingers, gently loosen the skin from the chicken breasts, thighs and drumsticks; try not to tear the skin.

5. Season the cavity of the chicken with salt and pepper and put the chicken in a roasting pan.

6. Using a small spoon, pour all but 1 tablespoon of the seasoning mixture under the skin of the chicken, rubbing it into the breasts, thighs and drumsticks.

7. Rub the butter under the skin of the breast meat.

8. Rub the remaining 1 tablespoon of the seasoned oil all over the chicken and season it with salt.

9. Put the reserved lemon halves in the cavity of the chicken and tie the legs together with twine.

10. Roast the chicken for about 1 1/2 hours, or until the juices from the cavity run clear and the chicken is browned and crisp.

11. Let the chicken rest in the roasting pan for 15 minutes.

12. Tilt the chicken to drain the juices from the cavity into the pan; transfer the chicken to a carving board.

13. Pour the pan juices into a bowl and skin the fat from the surface.

14. Strain the juice into a small saucepan and keep warm over low heat.

15. Carve the chicken and serve with the pan juices.

Cauliflower Alfredo Sauce with Spaghetti

Prepartion time

45 minutes

Ingredients

- 1 cauliflower
- 3 clove garlic crushed/you can also add roasted garlic when blending
- 2 Tbsp olive oil
- 1/2 tsp italian herb blend
- 2 tsp red pepper flakes or to taste
- salt and fresh ground pepper to taste
- 4 c water or chicken broth (broth is best)
- 1/4-1/2 c heavy cream
- 1/2 c grated parmesan cheese for topping

- 1/2 c fine bread crumbs
- 1/3 c grated parmesan cheese
- 1 Tbsp olive oil to taste
- 2 Tbsp any chopped fresh herbs (thyme, parsley, oregano, basil, etc.
- 14 oz box spaghetti, cooked and drained

Instructions

1. Cook and stir garlic cloves and 2 tbs olive oil in a large pot over medium heat until lightly browned and fragrant, 2-3 minutes.
2. Add cauliflower, water, Italian herbs, red pepper flakes, salt, and black pepper to taste.

3. Bring broth to a boil, cover, and cook until cauliflower is tender, about 10 min.

4. Meanwhile, combine bread crumbs, 1/3 cup parmesan cheeses, and 1 tbs olive oil in a skillet over medium heat; cook and stir until cheese has melted and mixture is browned, 2-3 minutes.

5. Turn off heat, sprinkle with salt to taste, and mix in basil' set aside.

6. Add cream to cauliflower mixture and puree in the pot with a stick blender or a food processor until smooth and creamy.

7. Stir in 2/3 cup parmesan cheese until melted; season with freshly ground black pepper to taste.

8. Mix in lemon juice with spaghetti and stir in alfredo sauce to coat pasta.

9. Serve topped with a sprinkle of parmesan cheese and the seasoned bread crumb mixture.

10. You can use any fresh herb in place of basil, such as thyme, parsley, or oregano. Or just sprig all of them.

Stuffed French Toast

Prepartion time

20 minutes

Ingredients

- bread slices
- 6 large eggs
- 1/4 c orange juice
- 2 Tbsp brown sugar
- 1 tsp vanilla extract
- 1 tsp cinnamon
- 1/2 tsp fresh ground nutmeg
- 2 pkg cream cheese, 8 oz each
- 1 stick butter
- 1 c confectioners' sugar
- 1 c chopped fresh strawberries

Instructions

For egg dip:

1. In a medium size bowl, slightly beat eggs, add orange juice, brown sugar, vanilla, cinnamon and nutmeg, mix well.

2. Set aside.

For filling:

1. In a medium-size mixing bowl beat together softened cream cheese, butter, confectioner sugar until well blended, add chopped strawberries and mix well.

2. Set aside.

3. Heat a non-stick skillet, add enough oil to coat bottom of the pan (about 1 tbsp).

4. Dip slices of bread in egg dip, fry on both sides till slightly browned.

5. Place one slice on plate plop 2 tbsp (or more) of filling onto it.

6. Top with another slice of french toast.

7. Sprinkle with confectioner sugar, top with whipped cream, fresh sliced strawberries and a little drizzle of syrup. Serve

2-Hour Turkey

Prepartion time

1 hour 30 minutes

Ingredients

- 1 thawed, whole turkey (from 10 - 24 pounds)
- 2 Tbsp olive oil, extra virgin
- 1 to 3 tsp coarsely ground salt (Kosher or sea)
- freshly ground pepper

Instructions

1. PREHEAT OVEN TO 475 degrees F (240-250 degrees C). This is what you'll roast it at for the ENTIRE time. Since this employs the use of a VERY hot oven, make sure your oven is CLEAN before you start, AND put about 1 inch of water in the bottom of the roasting pan to reduce the risk of smoking your family out of the house.

2. Remove all giblets, neck, pop-up thermometer (if there is one), and any trussing (like the

plastic thing that holds the legs together). Rinse turkey THOROUGHLY, inside and out with cool water, letting all water drain out of neck and body cavities. Pat dry, inside and out, with paper towels.

3. Place on V or U-shaped wire rack in roasting pan, so that turkey doesn't rest on the bottom of the pan. The first time I made this I didn't have a rack, so I just slapped it in my grandmother's old-fashioned blue-enamel roaster pan and it turned out FINE. If you don't have a rack...take a long piece of aluminum foil and wad it up into a long rope, then coil it in the bottom of the pan and rest your turkey on that.

4. Rub the entire outside of dried-off turkey with olive oil. Sprinkle generously with salt and

pepper. I use Kosher salt because it has large, coarse grains.

5. Pull wing tips AWAY from the body, twist them and tuck them, backward, under the bird... up by its neck.

6. Using aluminum foil, form caps over the end of each drumstick. If any parts of the turkey extend beyond the pan rim, make a foil "collar" underneath to make sure drippings flow back into the pan. Do NOT tie legs together, do NOT add stuffing, do NOT close body cavity. It's probably okay to put a little seasoning in the cavity (herbs, lemon, onion) but don't fill up the cavity.

7. Pour 2 inches of water into the bottom of the pan.

8. Bake on the 2nd to lowest rack in the oven.

9. Halfway through cooking time, turn the roasting pan around 180 degrees to ensure even cooking. Do NOT flip the bird over.

10. It's done when the internal temp (in the thickest part of BOTH the THIGH and BREAST is 160 degrees. Make certain they are BOTH at temp. Sometimes the thighs take a bit longer. When done, remove from the oven.

11. Cover completely with foil and let rest 30-45 minutes before carving. The internal temp will continue to rise to the recommended 165 degrees.

12. After resting, transfer to a platter for carving.

Best Fudge Brownie Mix

Prepartion time

30 minutes

Ingredients

FOR THE MIX

- 3 c all-purpose flour
- 2 tsp baking powder
- 2 tsp salt
- 4 c sugar
- 1/2 c unsweetened cocoa

FOR THE BROWNIES

- 2 1/2 c brownie mix
- 2 eggs, lightly beaten
- 1 tsp vanilla extract
- 1/2 c vegetable oil
- 1/4 c water

Instructions

1. To make the brownie mix: In a large bowl, sift together flour, baking powder and salt.

2. Add in sugar and cocoa.

3. Blend well, until evenly distributed.

4. Place mix in an air tight container and store in a cool, dry place. This mix will keep for a long time!

5. For the brownies: Preheat the oven to 350 degrees.

6. Spray an 8x8 pan with cooking spray.

7. In a medium bowl, combine 2 1/2 cups brownie mix with oil, eggs, vanilla and water and wisk together with a fork until dry ingredients are moistened.

8. Pour into a square pan and spread evenly. Bake at 350 for 25 minutes or until done in the center.

9. Double the brownie recipe for a 9x13 pan and bake for 28-30 minutes.

Marmalade Cream Cheese Coffee Cake

Prepartion time

1 hour 30 minutes

Ingredients

THE DOUGH

- Pam
- 3 canned buttermilk biscuits (not Grands)

THE FILLING

- 6 oz cream cheese
- 1/2 c sugar
- 1/4 c orange marmelade

THE COATING

- 4 Tbsp butter or magarine
- 1/2 c orange marmalade
- 1 c sugar

THE GLAZE

- 1 c powdered sugar
- 3 Tbsp orange juice
- the leftover marmalade and butter

Instructions

1. Preheat oven to 350. Spray a bundt pan with Pam.
2. Combine all ingredients for filling and beat until smooth.

3. Melt butter in a microwave safe dish and add marmalade to this. Microwave for about 30 seconds to melt marmalade.

4. Cool 2-3 minutes, stir frequently.

5. Put 1 cup of sugar in a shallow bowl.

6. Set up your workstation. A cutting board to prepare the biscuit. The bowl with the cream cheese, the bowl with the sugar, the bowl with the melted marmalade and butter.

7. Take a biscuit, flatten it and put a small dollop of the cream cheese mix in the middle.

8. Then fold in half pinching ends together. This is like making a stuffed dumpling or a pierogi or a ravioli. If you are having trouble with the cream cheese coming out, use less in the next biscuit.

9. Lightly dip folded biscuit into marmalade and butter mixture.

10. Then roll gently in the sugar mixture to lightly coat.

11. Put into pan with the seamed edge up. They should be laid next to each other like spoke on a bicycle wheel.

12. Repeat until all stuffed and rolled biscuits are in pan evenly layered.

13. Bake at 350 degrees for 30 minutes, the top will be browned.

14. While it's baking combine 1 cup of sugar, the remaining butter and marmalade mixture and 3 tablespoons of orange juice in a pan and bring to a simmer, stirring constantly.

15. When cake is done remove from oven and immediately invert onto a plate.

16. Spoon the glaze over all. This tastes good both warm and cold. Enjoy.

Hamburger, Sausage, Broccoli Alfredo - Low Carb

Prepartion time

1 hour 5 minutes

Ingredients

- 1 lb ground beef
- 1 lb bulk sausage (breakfast or Italian will work)

- 1 tsp oregano, dried
- 1 small onion, chopped
- 1 clove garlic, minced
- 10-12 oz fresh broccoli
- 1 pkg cream cheese, 8 oz.
- 1/2 c heavy cream
- 1/2 c Parmesan cheese, grated
- 8 oz mozzarella cheese, shredded
- salt and pepper, to taste

Instructions

1. In a large skillet, brown hamburger, sausage, onion, and garlic over a medium heat.

2. Season to taste with oregano, salt, and pepper; drain excess fat.

3. Meanwhile, steam the broccoli until tender yet still a little crisp; season with salt and pepper.

4. Place cream cheese in a microwaveable bowl and microwave on HIGH for about 45 seconds, until soft.

5. Whisk until creamy and smooth.

6. Gradually whisk in the cream until smooth; stir in the Parmesan cheese.

7. Combine hamburger, broccoli and cream sauce in a large greased casserole dish (2 ½ quart or larger).

8. Taste test and add additional salt, and pepper if desired.

9. Top with shredded cheese.

10. Bake at 350º for about 35-45 minutes, until bubbly around edges.

Yummy Chicken

Prepartion time

55 minutes

Ingredients

- 2 lb chicken boneless, skinless
- 1 pkg dry ranch dressing mix
- 1 c Parmesan cheese

- 1/2 c Corn Flakes, crushed
- 1/2 c butter, melted

Instructions

1. In a medium bowl, mix together ranch dressing mix, Parmesan cheese, and Corn Flakes.

2. Dip chicken in butter.

3. Then in mixture.

4. Place on a greased pan.

5. Bake at 375 for 40-50 minutes.

6. Enjoy!

Eggplant Parmesan

Prepartion time

50 minutes

Ingredients

- 1 eggplant, sliced 1/4-inch to 1/2-inch thick
- 6 eggs
- 2 c Italian bread crumbs
- 2 c Panko crumbs
- 1/2 c olive oil
- 1 Tbsp Italian seasoning
- 2 tsp garlic salt
- 1 - 2 c marinara sauce

- angel hair pasta
- 1/2 - 1 c frozen peas
- 5 - 6 Tbsp freshly grated Parmesan cheese
- 3 Tbsp freshly shredded mozzarella cheese

Instructions

1. Preheat oven to 350°F. In a large pot, fill halfway with water and bring to a boil.

2. While water is warming, heat a large skillet to medium-high heat and add oil.

3. Using 1 large bowl and 2 plates, set up a prepping station to bread the eggplant.

4. Crack eggs in a bowl and whisk well.

5. Place the Italian bread crumbs on one plate and place the Panko on the other plate.

6. Add Italian seasoning and garlic salt to the Panko and blend with a dry fork.

7. Working in batches, dip the eggplant slices in the egg (letting excess drip off).

8. Then coat with the Italian bread crumbs.

9. Back to the egg (letting excess drip off).

10. Then dip into the Panko crumbs.

11. Place the breaded eggplant slices in the skillet. Do not overcrowd the skillet.

12. Let the eggplant cook for about 2 minutes (or until brown) before flipping them over to the other side.

13. Let them get just a light golden brown.

14. Once the eggplant has been “seared” on both sides, place on a baking sheet lined with aluminum foil and lightly sprayed with non-stick cooking spray in a single layer.

15. Bake them for approximately 20 minutes.

16. While the eggplant is in the oven, warm the marinara sauce on medium-low heat. You may want to make sure this is covered with a lid to help prevent splattering.

17. Generously salt the boiling water and place the pasta in the boiling water in the other pot.

18. Cook pasta according to package. (You may want to start the pasta within the last 10-13 minutes of the cook time for the eggplant so everything stays nice and hot.)

19. During the last two minutes of the cook time for the pasta, add the peas.

20. Drain the pasta and peas using a colander.

21. Place drained pasta back in the pot.

22. Add about 3 tablespoons (or more) of the marinara sauce to the pasta and mix.

23. Place pasta and peas on a plate and top with the eggplant.

24. Add the marinara over top of the eggplant.

25. Add about 1-2 teaspoons of shredded Parmesan cheese and shredded mozzarella.

5 Cheese Macaroni

Prepartion time

50 minutes

Ingredients

- 1 box elbow macaroni, 16 ounces
- 1 stick butter
- 1 c shredded Muenster cheese
- 1 c shredded cheddar cheese
- 1 c shredded extra sharp cheddar cheese
- 1 c shredded Monterey Jack cheese
- 8 oz cubed processed cheese food (Velveeta)
- 1 1/2 c half-and-half
- 2 eggs
- 1/4 tsp salt

- 1/8 tsp ground black pepper

Instructions

1. Bring a large pot of water to a boil.
2. Add the pasta and cook for 8 to 10 minutes or until al dente; drain well and return to the cooking pot.
3. Add the stick of butter and mix it into the macaroni evenly.
4. In a large bowl, combine the Muenster cheese, mild and sharp cheddar cheeses, Monterey Jack cheese and processed cheese; combine cheeses well.
5. Then add it to the noodles.
6. Mix well.

7. Preheat oven to 350 degrees F (175 degrees C). In a small bowl, combine the half and half, eggs and salt and pepper. Mix this thoroughly.

8. Pour this into the noodle and cheese dish. Be sure to coat all of the noodles and cheese with the half and half mixture.

9. Transfer to a lightly greased deep 2 1/2 quart casserole dish or 9x13 pan.

10. Bake in preheated oven for 35 minutes or until hot and bubbling around the edges.

11. Serve and ENJOY!!!

Cream Cheese Stuffed Shells

Prepartion time

1 hour 25 minutes

Ingredients

- 3/4 box macaroni, large shells
- 2 pkg cream cheese
- 1 jar(s) prego traditional spaghetti sauce
- 1 bunch green onions
- 1 pkg mozzarella cheese

Instructions

1. pre-heat oven to 350 cook shells till al dente about 13 min in boiling water with a pinch of salt. grab a 5x9 cake pan line the bottom with a little less then half the spaghetti sauce.

2. Take cream cheese and mash it in a bowl then add the cut green onions.

3. set aside .

4. Wait for noodles to get done then drain and run under cold water till cool enough to handle then by spoonful add cream cheese mix to shells place open side down into spaghetti sauce in pan.

5. when finished filling shells top with the rest of spaghetti sauce and mozzarella cheese!

6. Place in oven till mozzarella cheese starts to brown about 25 min take out and serve! goes great with a salad and bread sticks.

The Original "Easiest Pineapple Cake"

Prepartion time

45 minutes

Ingredients

- 2 c all-purpose flour
- 2 c sugar
- 2 eggs
- 1 tsp baking soda

- 1 tsp vanilla
- 1 pinch salt
- 1 can(s) crushed pineapple (undrained) in its own juice - not syrup, 20 oz.
- 1 c chopped nuts, optional

CREAM CHEESE FROSTING

- 1/2 c butter or 1 stick
- 1 pkg cream cheese, softened, 8 oz.
- 1 tsp vanilla
- 1 1/2 c confectioners' sugar
- shredded coconut for garnish, optional

Instructions

1. Preheat oven to 350 degrees F.

2. Put all the cake ingredients into a large mixing bowl.

3. Mix all of the cake ingredients together.

4. Pour into a greased 9X13 inch pan.

5. Bake at 350 for 35 - 40 minutes (until the top is golden brown).

6. For the frosting: Beat butter, cream cheese and vanilla together until creamy.

7. Gradually mix in powdered sugar.

Twice Baked Potato Casserole

Prepartion time

1 hour 5 minutes

Ingredients

- 8 potatoes, peeled and cut into quarters (about 3 pounds)
- 1/2 c butter
- 1/2 c sour cream
- salt & pepper
- 1 pkg bacon, chopped & fried crisp
- 2 c sharp cheddar cheese, divided
- 1/4 c heavy cream
- 4 oz cream cheese

Instructions

1. Boil potatoes in salted water. Cook until tender.

2. Drain potatoes and place into mixing bowl. Add cream cheese, sour cream, butter, cream, salt, and pepper. Continue mixing until smooth.

3. Fold in 1 cup of the cheese and half the bacon.

4. Pour into a 3 qt baking dish.

5. Bake for 15 minutes at 350.

6. Top with remaining cheese and bacon. Bake for an additional 15 minutes to melt the cheese.

7. Remove from the oven and garnish with chopped green onions if desired.

Roast Sticky Chicken Rotisserie Style Like the Deli

Prepartion time

26 hours

Ingredients

- 1 whole chicken, 4 - 5 pounds
- 4 tsp salt
- 2 tsp paprika
- 1 tsp onion powder
- 1 tsp thyme, dried

- 1 1/2 tsp black pepper
- 1 tsp cayenne pepper
- 1/2 tsp garlic powder
- 2 large onions
- cooking oil to rub chicken

Instructions

1. In a small bowl, mix together salt, paprika, onion powder, thyme, pepper, cayenne pepper, and garlic powder.

2. Remove and discard giblets from chicken. Rinse chicken cavity and pat dry with paper towel.

3. Rub chicken with oil then inside and out and under the skin with spice mixture.

4. Place 1 onion into each cavity of the chicken.

5. Place chicken in a resealable bag or double wrap with plastic wrap. Refrigerate overnight, or at least 4 to 6 hours.

6. Preheat oven to 325 degrees F (120 degrees C). Place chicken in a roasting pan. Bake uncovered for 1 1/2 - 2 hours, to a minimum internal temperature of 180 degrees F (85 degrees C). Use meat thermometer to check in the thigh.

7. Baste a few times the last hour if not using a rotisserie.

8. Let the chicken stand, covered in foil, for 10 minutes.

9. Then carve.

My Favorite Loaded Potato Soup

Prepartion time

1 hour

Ingredients

- 1/2 stick butter
- 1 small onion, diced
- 2 medium carrots, diced about the same size as onion

- 2-3 clove garlic, minced (My family loves garlic so I add 3-4 cloves. Add however much you like.)
- 2 Tbsp all-purpose flour
- 8 medium russet potatoes, peeled and cubed
- 4 c milk, whole, 2% or 1%
- 2 chicken bouillon cubes
- 1 c half and half
- 1 1/2 tsp salt
- 1/2 tsp pepper
- bacon bits, for garnish
- grated cheddar cheese, for garnish

Instructions

1. In a large saucepan, melt the butter and saute the onion, garlic, and carrots until both are slightly tender (about 5 minutes).

2. Whisk in the flour and cook for 1 minute.

3. Add the milk and drop bouillon cube in to dissolve.

4. Add the potatoes. Cook over medium heat for 15 minutes until the potatoes are very soft and some of them have begun to dissolve into mush.

5. Add the half and half, salt, and pepper. (May need more salt; add to taste). Simmer on the stove over medium-low heat for 25 min or until nice and hot.

6. Serve soup sprinkled with bacon bits and grated cheese.

Hearty Lasagna for Two

Prepartion time

1 hour 10 minutes

Ingredients

DADS PERFECT SAUCE

- 3/4 lb ground beef

- 1/2 lb ground turkey sausage, or sweet sausage
- 1/2 c chopped onion
- 2 clove smashed garlic with peel off
- 1 can(s) crushed tomatoes (28oz)
- 1 can(s) tomato paste (12oz)
- 1 can(s) tomato sauce (15oz)
- 1/2 c water
- 2 Tbsp sugar
- 1 1/2 tsp dried basil leaves
- 1/2 tsp fennel seeds
- 1 tsp italian seasoning
- 3/4 Tbsp salt

- 1/4 tsp pepper
- 1 tsp dried parsley

CHEESE MIX

- 8 oz ricotta cheese
- 1 large egg
- 1/4 tsp salt
- 1 tsp dried parsley

ADDITIONAL INGREDIENTS

- 6 lasagna noodles, rinsed with warm water
- 1 pkg mozzarella cheese/provolone cheese mix shredded or sliced (2 cups shredded)

- 1/4 c plus 2 tbsp of parmesan cheese.

Instructions

1. In Crock pot, cook meat, onion and garlic on a high temp until meat starts to brown and onions and garlic have sweated, but not burned.

2. Stir in crushed tomatoes, paste, sauce and water.

3. Season with sugar, basil, fennel seeds, Italian seasoning, 3/4 tbsp salt, pepper and 1 tsp of dried parsley.

4. Let this come up in temperature, cover and simmer for approx 2 1/2 hrs.

5. Prepare noodles by breaking noodles to fit an 8x8 baking pan. Set aside until ready to assemble after sauce has simmered.

6. Once it has simmered long enough, turn off Crock pot rinse the noodles with warm water, no need to cook the noodles.

7. Preheat oven to 375° F.

8. Prepare cheese mixture by adding ricotta cheese, egg, 1 tsp parsley and 1/4 tsp salt.

9. Add 1 tbsp of the Parmesan cheese and mix to combine.

10. To Assemble: With a 1/2 c measuring cup, or ladle, place one or 1 1/2 scoops of sauce on the bottom of the 8x8 pan.

11. Place one layer of your pre-measured noodles on the sauce.

12. Spread or dollop the ricotta mixture on top of the noodles and try to spread it best you can.

13. Sprinkle or place the Mozzarella/Provolone cheese mixture on top of that.

14. Next, another layer of the sauce, then sprinkle the Parmesan cheese over that. You repeat this (starting with another layer of noodles) until all of the ricotta is gone. I did two good layers with about 1-1 1/2 cups sauce in each layer, and 2 hand fulls of the shredded cheese mix, to give you an idea.

15. Once you have completed the last layer with Parmesan, I sprinkle a little extra, if any, of the shredded cheese on there too.

16. Cover this tight with foil. PLACE ON BAKING SHEET, this probably will bubble over slightly. Into the 375° oven for 25 minutes.

17. Very carefully, remove the foil at this point, and continue to bake for an additional 25 minutes or so.

18. Remove from oven and let lasagna cool for 15 minutes or so.

19. Meanwhile, you can store the remaining sauce in a freezer container, make an additional lasagna (8x8 pretty aluminum pan, just be careful as it will be heavy, may want to use a baking sheet until the freezer sets it up) and freeze it for a later day or keep in the fridge for spaghetti, pizza, bread stick dipping sauce or whatever you want to use this for.

Quinoa Stuffed Mushrooms

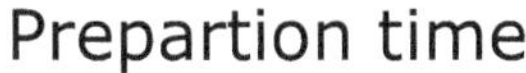

Prepartion time

3 hours

Ingredients

- 4-6 clove very finely minced garlic
- 1 large, finely chopped onion
- 1-2 stringed finely chopped celery ribs
- 1/4 small very finely chopped cabbage-use only the very inner part of the cabbage*
- 1/4 c minced fresh parsley leaves
- 3-4 * finely minced green onions
- 1/2 lb meatless crumbles*

- 2 crumbled Garden Veggie patties
- 1/2 tsp dry, crushed red pepper flakes
- 1/8 c chopped walnuts
- 3 tsp ground flax seed (opt.)
- to taste Zatarain's seasoning-spicy salt, sans the msg
- 1/2 bunch fresh, washed, and well drained baby spinach
- 1/8 c grated Parmesan cheese*
- 1 1/2 * fresh roasted red peppers
- 1 c quinoa, cooked with a bay leaf and 1 tbsp olive oil
- 1 pkg baby portebello mushrooms, with the stems removed

- dash(es) ground nutmeg and clove, to taste

Instructions

1. In a large stock pot, saute onions, garlic, celery, cabbage, and parsley until tender and a bit dry.

2. Add the meatless crumbles, and the crumbled veggie patty, walnuts, spices, and the cooked quinoa.

3. Mix gently and set aside.

4. Coat the bottom of a large baking pan with olive oil.

5. Tear the cooled red peppers into strips. (Each pepper should yield eight strips).

6. Lay eight strips down on the bottom of the baking pan.

7. Spread the spinach leaves on top of the red peppers.

8. Sprinkle the cheese on top of the spinach.

9. Place the mushrooms on top, with the hole side up.

10. Cover everything with the quinoa mix, making sure that the caps are nice and full of the mix.

11. Lay the remaining strips of red peppers on top of the mix.

12. Bake at 350 for about 50 min.

13. There are several ways that you can roast peppers. The 'laziest' way is to put a sheet of

parchment paper on a baking tray, spray the pepper with cooking spray and set the oven to 350.

14. Put the peppers in, uncovered for about 45 minutes. When the peppers are about half done, turn them over. The skin is very hot!! When the pepper is exposed to air, and the skin peels away easily, it is done.

15. Remove from the oven, and cover with a big bowl (to allow them to steam).

16. After they cool, the skin will slip right off of them. You can also broil the peppers. I stand right next to my oven when I use this method, as the peppers burn very quickly. This method only takes about ten minutes, but be sure that all sides are darkened.

17. Follow above directions after removing the peppers from the oven. The third way is done on the stove using a hot skillet.

18. Just roll the peppers back and forth until they are blackened.

19. Another way is to stick a fork in the pepper, hold over a gas flame until blackened.

20. Follow as above. Or, you can pick up a jar of them from the grocery.

21. I like to use the inner 'chunk' of cabbage since it is much sweeter. It is ok to use all of the green onion, white as well as green. My meatless brand of choice is Morning Star. Both the crumbles and the Garden Veggie patties can be found in the freezer section, in green packaging. The patties will add an extra bit of crunch, as

they have water chestnuts in them. If you choose to use the flax seed, it doesn't change the taste the, but it will thicken the entire dish. I was going to use mozzarella cheese but was out. The Parmesan cheese worked fine. I wasn't going for a binder since the flax seed will do that.

Enchilada Stuffed Shells

Prepartion time

45 minutes

Ingredients

- 15-20 jumbo pasta shells
- 1 lb ground beef or turkey
- 2 (10 oz) cans enchilada sauce
- 1/2 tsp dried minced onion
- 1/4 tsp oregano, dried
- 1/4 tsp basil, dried
- 1/4 tsp ground cumin
- 1/2 c refried beans
- 1 c colby and jack cheese, shredded

Instructions

1. Preheat oven to 350 degrees. Cook pasta shells according to package directions. Drain and set aside.

2. Make sure thy are separated so they do not stick together.

3. In a large skillet over medium heat, brown the ground beef until no longer pink. Drain the fat.

4. Stir in minced onion, oregano, basil and cumin.

5. Stir one cup of the enchilada sauce into the meat mixture.

6. Stir in the refired beans and set aside.

7. Fill each cooked pasta shell with the beef mix.

8. Coat an 9x13 inch baking dish with non stick spray and pour half of the remaining can of enchilada sauce evenly over the bottom.

9. Place each stuffed shell into the baking dish and pour the remaining half of the enchilada sauce over the tops of the shells with the meat mix.

10. Cover and bake for 20 minutes then remove dish from oven and sprinkle the jack cheese on top of the shells.

11. Bake another 5 minutes until the cheese melts.

12. Serve and enjoy.

Crock Pot Cheesy Scalloped Potatoes and Ham

Prepartion time

4 hours 15 minutes

Ingredients

- 10 medium Idaho potatoes; peeled
- 8 oz pkg diced ham, or cut your own
- 1/2 c chopped onion (I use frozen-no more tears!!)
- 1 can(s) Campbell's cheddar cheese soup
- 1 can(s) cream of mushroom soup, light
- 1 /2 c cheddar cheese, shredded
- 1 tsp dry mustard and white pepper

KICKED UP CREAMY VERSION

- 2 Tbsp butter or margarine
- 4 Tbsp flour
- 1 can(s) fat free evaporated milk
- 1-1 1/2 c shredded swiss cheese
- paprika, just a sprinkle

Instructions

Regular version:

1. In a large bowl mix the two soups and feel free to add a tiny splash of milk, then add the onion, hams and seasonings.

2. Slice the potatoes in half and then into slices; add to soup and mix well.

3. Put into the crock pot, and add a sprinkle of paprika.

4. Cook on high 4 hours or low 7-8 hours.

5. Sprinkle the cheddar on top during last 10 min.

Kicked Up version:

1. Place peeled potatoes in a bowl of water.

2. Melt the butter over med-high heat, cook and stir a few mins.

3. Then whisk in the flour and stir.

4. Add 1 cup of the evaporated milk and stir over med-high heat until bubbly and thickened; you may need the whole can.

5. Stir in the cheddar soup, Swiss and cheddar cheese and seasonings, stir till melted and creamy. (You will not use the mushroom soup in this version :)

6. Slice potatoes in half and then into slices.

7. Place in a large bowl, along with onions and ham; mix well.

8. Place in crock pot and cook the same as regular version. Let stand 10 min prior to serving.

9. Some people like to layer the ingredients, instead of mixing in a bowl. I like it all mixed so the flavors marry. Use your preference!

Chicken Alfredo

Prepartion time

50 minutes

Ingredients

- 4 boneless chicken breasts
- 1 lb rotini (1 box)
- 2 jar(s) Ragu roasted garlic parmesan cheese sauce
- olive oil
- salt
- pepper

- 1 tsp parsley
- 1/3 c grated Parmesan cheese

Instructions

1. Boil the rotini in a large pot until done, approximately 8-12 minutes. Add salt to the water.

2. Clean and cube chicken.

3. In a large frying pan add a few teaspoons of olive oil and put burner on medium high.

4. Add the chicken.

5. When chicken is almost done add salt and pepper to taste and the parsley.

6. Drain the rotini when it is ready.

7. Place back into pot. Add the chicken and the Ragu.

8. Stir over low heat.

9. If you are making this dish for company add to a baking pan for presentation.

10. Top with Parmesan cheese and crisp in the oven on broil for about 5 minutes.

Biscuits & Gravy Breakfast Casserole

Prepartion time

45 minutes

Ingredients

- 10 oz tube of buttermilk biscuit dough
- 6 eggs
- 1 pkg powdered country gravy pouch (plus ingredients per package to make gravy)
- 1 lb sausage, any flavor
- 1 c cheese, shredded
- 1/2 c milk
- salt and pepper, to taste

Instructions

1. Preheat oven to 350. Take a 13x9-in pan and spray with cooking spray (or smear with butter).

2. Cut biscuit dough into 1" pieces, and line the bottom of the pan.

3. Brown the sausage & drain.

4. Scatter the browned sausage over the biscuit pieces, then top with shredded cheese.

5. Whisk eggs and milk with a pinch of salt and pepper, then pour over the pan.

6. Make gravy according to instructions, and pour over the pan. Bake for 30-45 minutes, depending how hot your oven runs.

7. Cut and serve. It's delicious warm right out of the oven!

Amazing "Date Night" Chicken Tacos

Prepartion time

1 hour 10 minutes

Instructions

FILLING:

- 3 Tbsp butter or margerine
- 1/2 c finely diced white onion
- 2 lb boneless, skinless chicken tenderloins
- 3 c water
- 16 oz Pace picante sauce (mild or medium** reserving 1/3 cup**)
- 1/2 tsp salt

- 1/2 tsp pepper
- 1/2 Tbsp adobo seasoning
- 1 Tbsp chopped fresh cilantro (fresh works best)

TOPPINGS:

- 1 Tbsp butter or margerine
- 1 pkg flour tortillas
- 2 c finely shredded iceburg lettuce
- 1/2 c fresh chopped cilantro
- 2 c shredded queso fresco or monterey jack cheese
- 1 1/2 c finely chopped tomatoes (optional)
- 1/2 c sour cream (optional)

Instructions

1. Start by heating butter over medium heat in a large (deep) frying pan or dutch oven. Saute the onions until almost caramelized (just a hint of color).

2. Then add the fresh chicken and cook until the chicken loses it's pink color and starts to SLIGHTLY brown..about 4-5 mins. (don't overcook or chicken will not end up tender)

3. Next add your water, dry spices and the jar of Pace Picante sauce (reserving the 1/3 c. for garnish later) turn heat up to medium/high, raising to a slow boil, and cook for about 45 mins (cover with lid to reduce evaporation of liquid!).

4. Check & stir frequently and add small amounts of water if needed (the chicken will be "stewing" and should have A LOT of liquid, so adjust your heat so that it doesn't dry out/scorch).

5. By this time, most of the liquid should be absorbed, but chicken mixture should be "saucy."

6. Take 2 forks and begin to shred all the chicken until it's the consistency you like

7. Stewing the chicken for so long creates a great soft/moist texture and really infuses the meat with all those wonderful flavors! Of course add a pinch of any of the dry seasonings to suit your personal taste :) Lastly, add the (1) tbsp of

butter to give the "sauce" a nice richness and finishing touch :)

8. Start assembling your tacos with a (warmed) tortilla shell filled with the stewed chicken, lettuce, fresh cilantro, cheese, tomatoes, the 1/3 c. reserved Picante, etc. These are fabulous Amazing "Date Night" Chicken Tacos with a side of refried beans and yellow (Saffron) rice.

Warm Ya up Chili

Prepartion time

30 minutes

Ingredients

- 3 lb ground chuck...any ground meat will do, i just skim the fat off
- 3 Tbsp minced garlic
- 1/4 c chili powder
- 1/2 tsp oregeno
- 2 tsp onion powder
- 2 Tbsp paprika
- 1 tsp cumin
- 1/2 tsp cayenne pepper
- 2 tsp salt...more if you like

- 1 tsp black pepper
- 15 oz can crushed tomatoes
- 15 oz can tomato sauce
- 15 oz red wine (any..can replace with water if not avail)
- 1 c water
- 2 Tbsp masa
- 2 Tbsp sugar

Instructions

1. In a large stock pot brown ground meat.
2. When the meat is cooking add seasonings.
3. When it is all good and brown add tomato sauce and wine then water.

4. Let cook down for a few minutes.

5. Add crushed tomatoes.

6. Bring up to a slow bubble for about 15 minutes..then add masa to thicken. Then add sugar to cut acid.

7. Bring up to a slow bubble for 10 mins or so.

8. Cover for 15 minutes and allow spices to mingle.

9. Serve by itself or with crackers, cornbread or over your favortie item.

Deli Roses

Prepartion time

30 minutes

Ingredients

- 1 package Gefen Puff Pastry, thawed
- 1 pound pastrami, thinly-sliced
- 1 cup Haddar Honey Mustard

Instructions

1. Preheat oven to 375 degrees Fahrenheit.

2. Lightly grease two twelve-cup muffin pans with oil.

3. On a lightly-floured work surface, roll out one piece of puff pastry to a 14 inch x20 inch rectangle.

4. Position the dough horizontally, facing you.

5. Using the Betty Bossi Rose Roller, cut the dough into six scalloped strips.

6. Brush honey mustard on the dough. Top with sliced pastrami. Brush with some more honey mustard.

7. Roll up the pastry and slice in half through the center of the roll so you have two roses.

8. Place "rose" in the muffin pan, scalloped side up. Repeat with remaining sheet of puff pastry.

9. Bake for 20 minutes or until dough is puffed and golden brown.

London Broil

Prepartion time

30 minutes

Ingredients

- 2 tablespoons Gefen Olive Oil
- 1 teaspoon salt
- 1/2 teaspoon pepper
- 1 teaspoon chili powder (or make your own)
- 1/2 tablespoon coffee granules, such as Haddar Instant Coffee
- 2 pounds (1 kilogram) London broil

Instructions

1. Set the oven to broil.
2. Place the London broil in a baking pan and rub with the olive oil and all of the spices.

3. Place in the oven directly under the broiler, making sure that your oven rack is as high as it can go.

4. Broil for three to five minutes on each side (depending on how strong your broiler is).

5. Remove the pan from the oven and reduce oven heat to 250 degrees Fahrenheit (120 degrees Celsius).

6. When the oven reaches this temperature, return the pan to the oven and bake for 15-20 minutes.

Crunchy Schnitzel with Veggie Chips

Prepartion time

30 minutes

Ingredients

- 12 slices thin chicken cutlets, about 2-3 pounds
- 4 tablespoons oil
- 4 large eggs
- 3/4 cup Manischewitz Potato Starch
- 1 and 1/2 teaspoons turmeric
- 1 and 1/2 teaspoons garlic powder
- 1/2 teaspoon ground ginger
- 3/4 teaspoon salt
- heaping 1/4 teaspoon black pepper
- 2 (5-ounce) bags Heaven and Earth Veggie Salad Toppers

- 1 cup Haddar Gluten-Free Japanese Style Panko crumbs

Instructions

1. Preheat oven to 450 degrees Fahrenheit.

2. Place two tablespoons oil on each of two jellyroll pans.

3. Use a pastry brush to coat the entire pan with oil. If you need to bake a third batch, add one tablespoon oil to the pan and then heat the pan.

4. Place the eggs into a shallow bowl and beat well.

5. Place the potato starch into another shallow bowl.

6. Add the turmeric, garlic powder, ginger, salt and pepper and mix well.

7. Place the veggie sticks into the bowl of a food processor and chop into very small pieces.

8. Place into a shallow bowl.

9. Add the panko and mix well.

10. Dip each piece of chicken into the potato starch to coat completely, shaking off excess, then into the beaten eggs, letting the excess drip off for at least 15 seconds, and then press into the crumb mixture to completely coat the chicken.

11. Place the pieces on a dinner plate once they are ready.

12. Line a cookie sheet with aluminum foil and place a cooling rack on top.

13. When the oven is preheated, place the oil-coated pans into the oven and heat for five minutes.

14. When the pans are hot, carefully remove one pan at a time and add the schnitzel pieces, without touching each other.

15. Place back into the oven and bake for ten minutes.

16. Turn over and bake for another five minutes.

17. Rotate the pans halfway through so each pan has a turn on the bottom rack.

18. Place baked schnitzel on the cooling rack to cool, to retain the maximum crunchiness, until serving.

Asian Beef Stir Fry Bowl Asian Beef Stir Fry Bowl

Prepartion time

30 minutes

Ingredients

- 3 tablespoons oil, divided
- 2 cups frozen broccoli cuts

- 3/4 pound ground beef
- 1 packet Heaven & Earth 3 Minute Brown Rice
- 1/4 cup brown sugar
- 1/4 cup Gefen Soy Sauce
- 2 tablespoons Gefen Sesame Oil

Instructions

1. Microwave rice for three or four minutes (depending on the strength of your microwave) according to package instructions.

2. Season with salt to taste.

3. Heat a sauté pan with one tablespoon of oil.

4. Add broccoli and sauté for a few minutes, until warmed through.

5. Season with salt to taste.

6. Add remaining oil to pan.

7. Add ground beef and cook, smashing with a large fork to brown.

8. Meat should be cooked in four to five minutes.

9. Stir together brown sugar, soy sauce, and sesame oil and stir into meat.

10. Assemble the bowl.

11. Add rice to the bottom and top with meat and broccoli.

12. Sprinkle with sesame seeds and scallions to garnish.

Easy Teriyaki Salmon

Prepartion time

30 minutes

Ingredients

- 2 salmon fillets
- 3 tablespoons oil
- 3 tablespoons Haddar Teriyaki Sauce
- 3 tablespoons Gefen Honey
- Gefen Garlic Powder
- sesame seeds

Instructions

For the Salmon

1. Preheat oven to 400°F.

2. Spray a baking pan with non-stick cooking spray.

3. Clean and dry salmon.

4. Lay salmon down in baking pan.

5. Drizzle the oil, teriyaki sauce, and honey on the top and smear.

6. Sprinkle the garlic powder and sesame seeds.

7. Bake uncovered for 20 minutes.

Broccoli Mini Kugels

Prepartion time

25 minutes

Ingredients

- 1 bag Beleaf Frozen Broccoli
- 1 bag cauliflower
- 4 eggs
- salt and pepper to taste

Instructions

Make the Kugels

1. Briefly steam lots of broccoli and cauliflower. Drain and mash.

2. Add eggs, salt, and pepper.

3. Bake in muffin tins sprayed with olive oil with a little oil drizzled on top at 350 degrees Fahrenheit for 15 minutes.

Oven Fried Cornflake Chicken

Prepartion time

1 hour 30 minutes

Ingredients

- 1 chicken, skinned and cut in eighths
- 1 cup flour

- 3 eggs
- 3 tablespoons Heaven & Earth Ketchup
- 1 cup Gefen Corn Flake Crumbs
- 1 teaspoon salt
- 1 teaspoon garlic powder
- 1 teaspoon Gefen Parsley Flakes
- oil

Instructions

1. Prepare three bowls to coat chicken.
2. Put flour in one bowl.
3. Combine eggs and ketchup in another bowl.

4. Combine corn flake crumbs and spices in a third bowl.

5. Prepare a 9x13-inch pan with 1/4 to 1/2 inch of oil.

6. Dredge chicken in flour, then eggs, and lastly with crumbs.

7. Place in pan, face-down.

8. Bake, uncovered, at 400 degrees Fahrenheit for 30 minutes.

9. Turn chicken over and bake another 30 minutes.

.

www.ingramcontent.com/pod-product-compliance
Ingram Content Group UK Ltd.
Pitfield, Milton Keynes, MK11 3LW, UK
UKHW022003190726
13853UKWH00004B/1710